The Cycle of
ADHD, Autism Spectrum Disorder, and Depression
An Individual Research

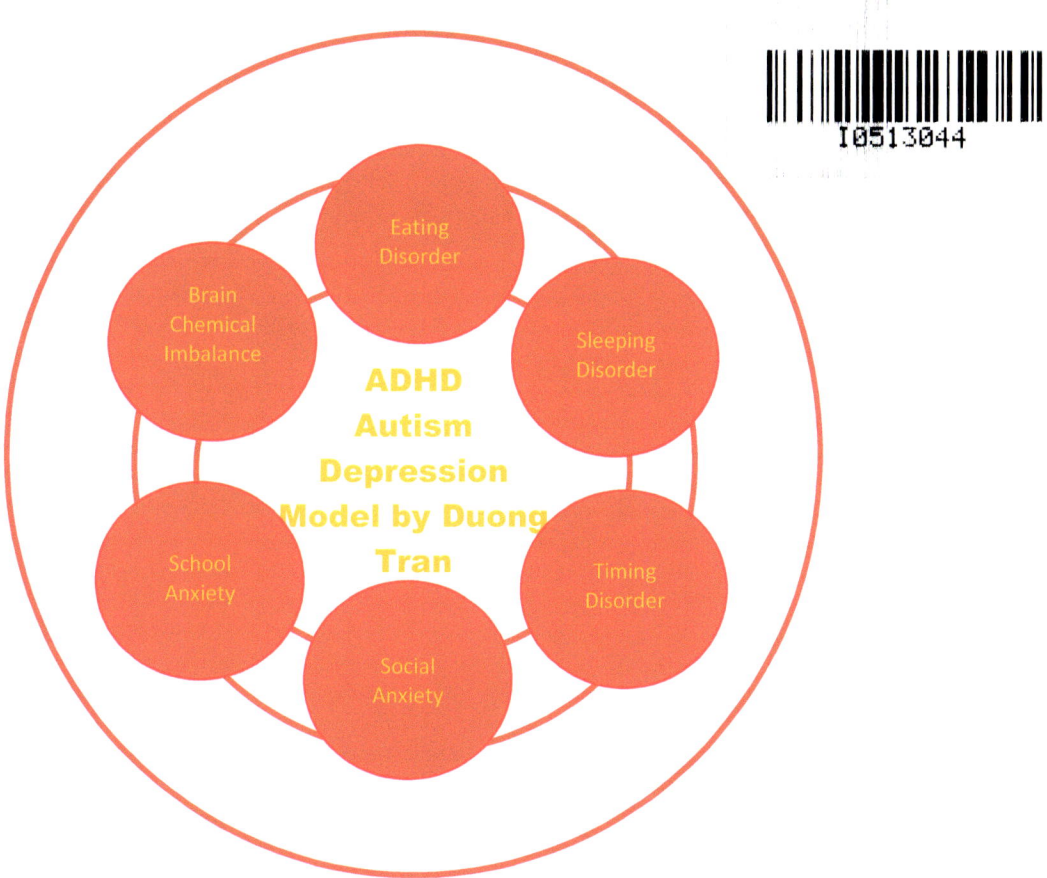

In my theory or visual knowledge, there is a one-two-three cycle spectrum disorder: ADHD, Autism, and Depression all-in-one. I created this model to discover the behaviors and the problems of my son.

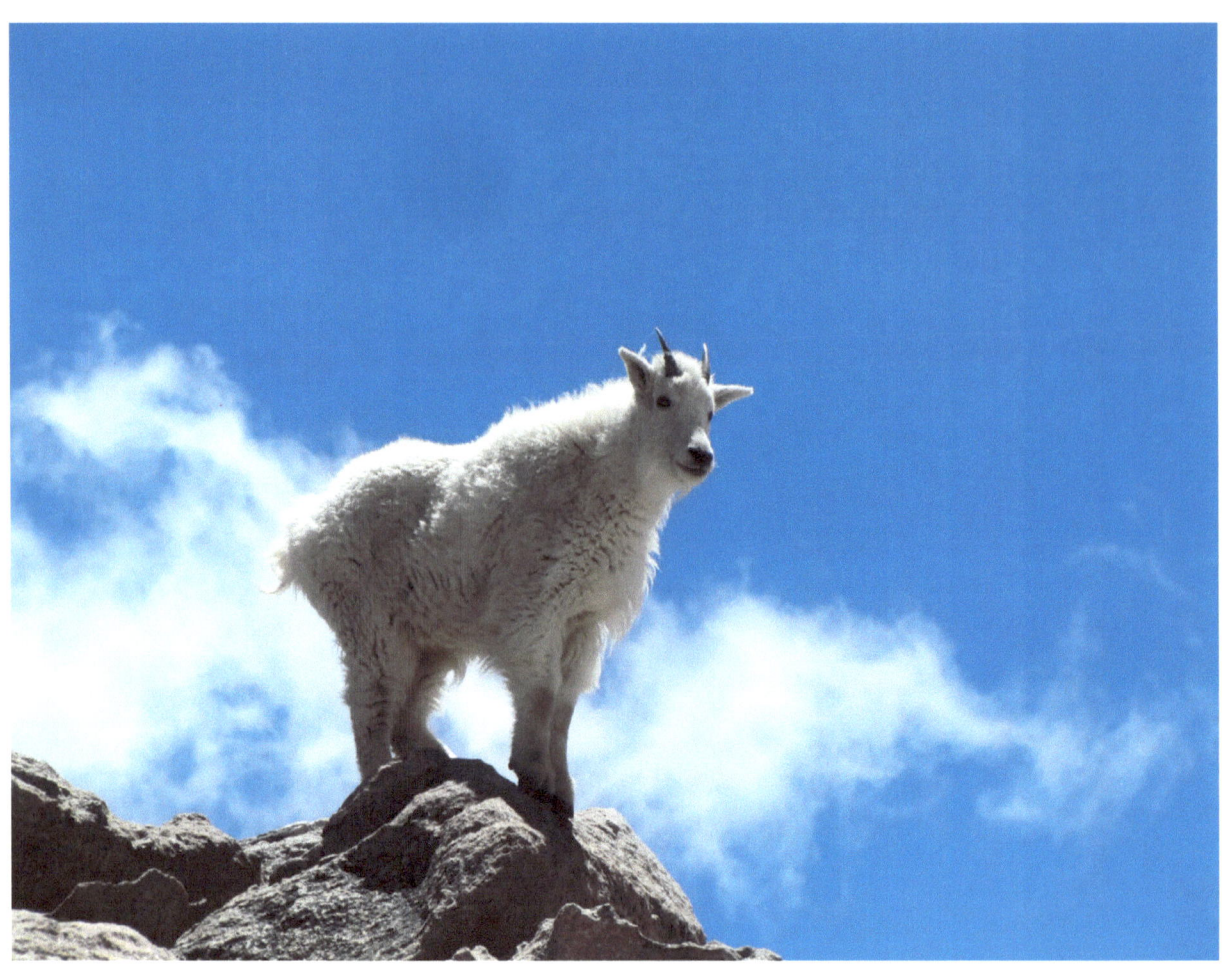

Dear Readers and Viewers, I choose the mountain goat to represent ADHD, autism spectrum disorder, and depression. The mountain goat is a loner, runner, hyperactive jumping, painless, head banging, looking like autism and depression.

This book is in individual study of ADHD, autism, and depression which contains the facts and a collection of information. The book includes my knowledge, research, and experience studying my son of having all ADHD, autism, and depression. I believe it will help other kids. Parents are the doctors, and the real doctors are experts to provide the medicines. There are treatments for all, ADHD, autism spectrum disorder and depression.

Thank you for buying multiple copies of my books and support me at
https://www.gofundme.com/f/cycleofautism

Copyrights: Book Cover, ideas, theories, words by Duong Tran.

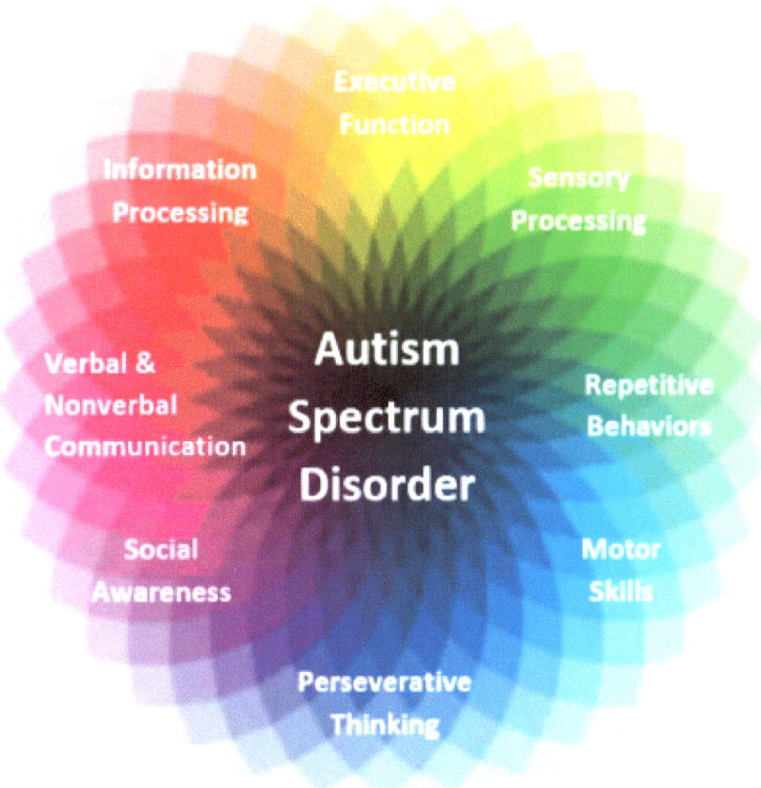

https://carmenbpingree.com/blog/what-is-autism-spectrum-disorder/

ADHD (Attention-deficit/hyperactivity disorder), autism, and depression signs begin at birth, 3 months old, 6 months old, 9 months old, 1 year old, 2 years old, 4 years old, or daily life behaviors. Mostly, repetitive behaviors, sensitive to difference food, sleeping problem, no attention, and not playing with other kids. Other signs include slow communication in either one or more family languages, hyperactive running and jumping. The head banging is a sign of both autism and depression. A child may have one or multiple symptoms.

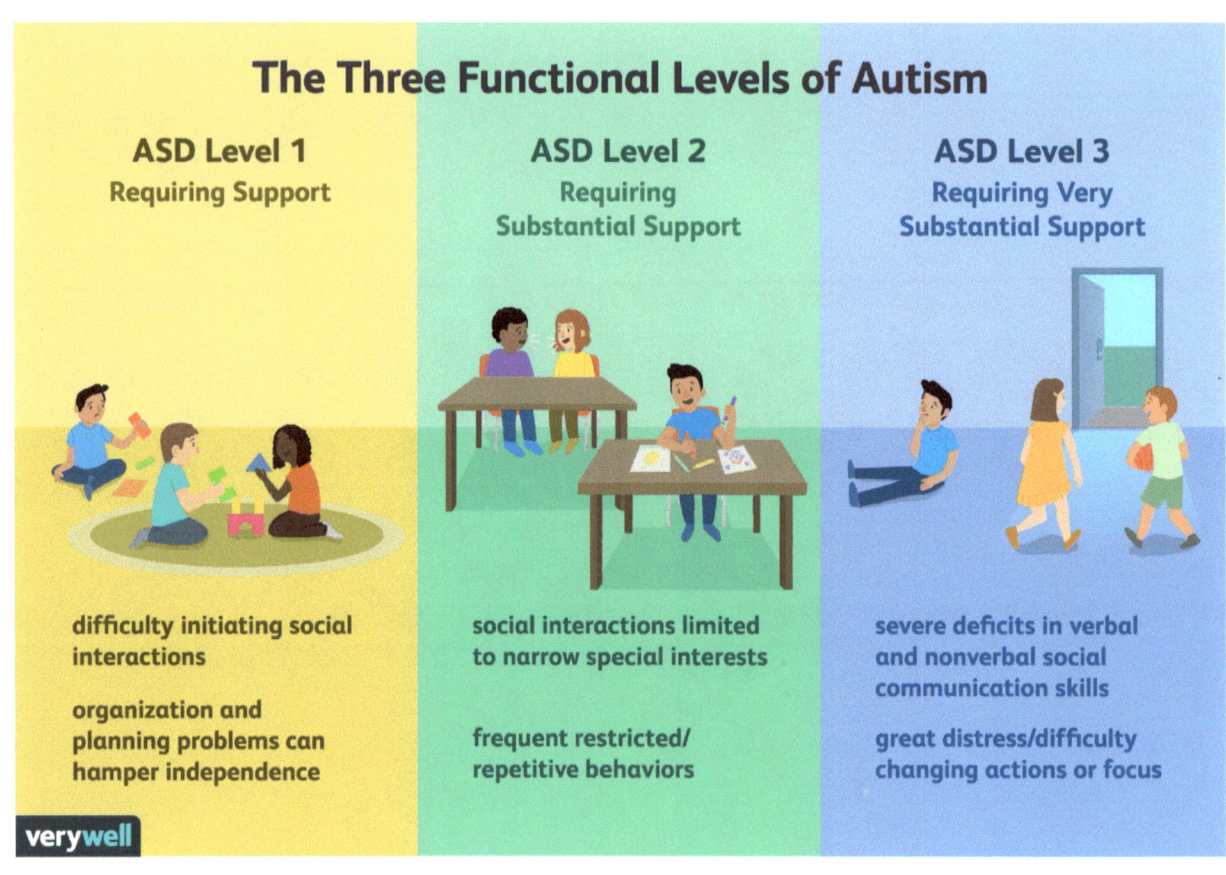

Understanding the Three Levels of Autism (verywellhealth.com)

There are three levels of autism as in the picture by professionals. Whatever, all levels are autism, and all autism have the same problems. Autism may lead to depression injuring bodies. Unlike autism and depression, ADHD kids are hyperactive and seem to be smart ones mean while autism may have hidden talents. The same for all needs to be cured.

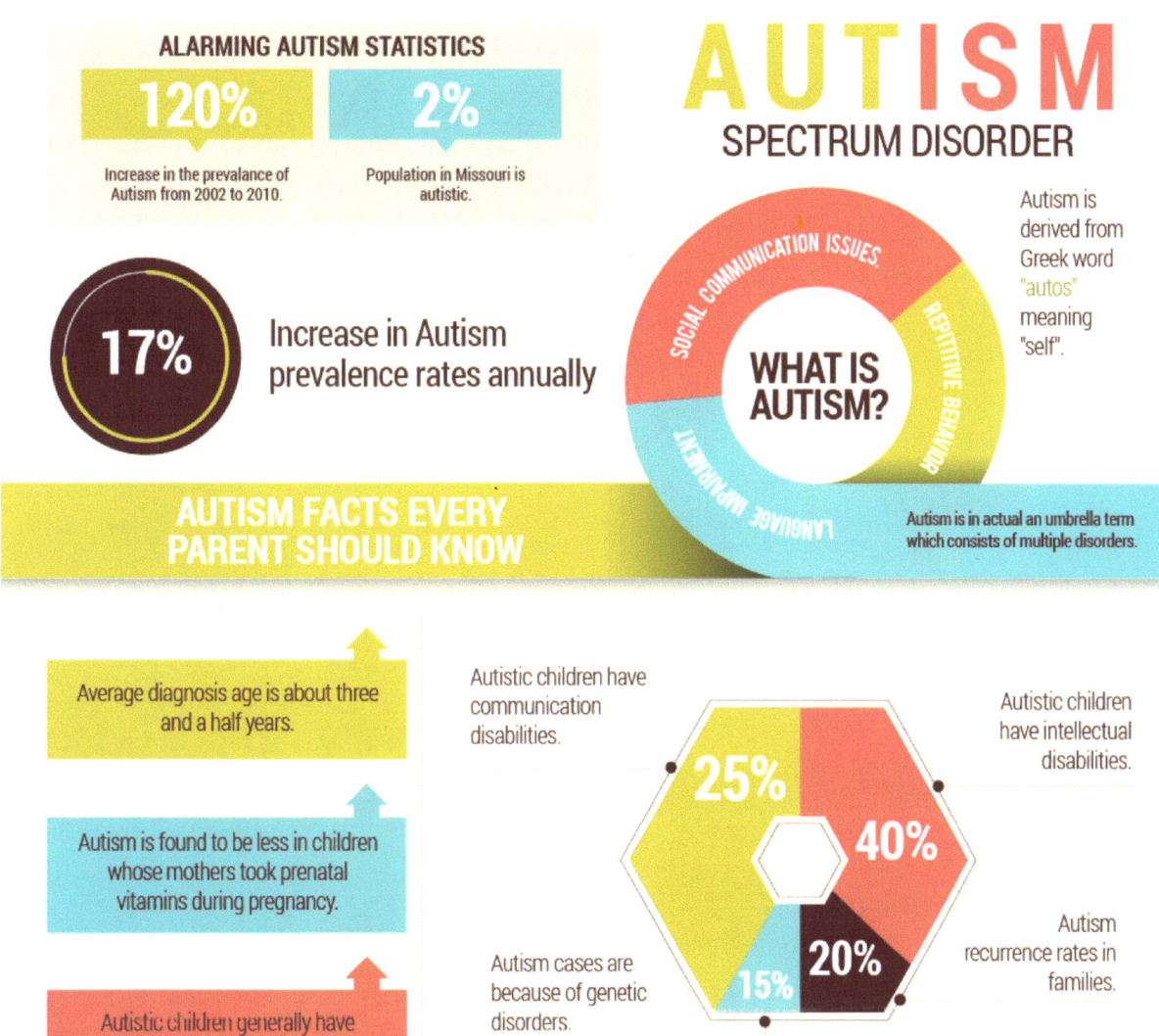

Due to the living disorder of our life, children with autism are increasing over the years. Children can be affected by parent genes or current life. Understanding the social life can help people to live better.

AUTISM SPECTRUM DISORDER (ASD)

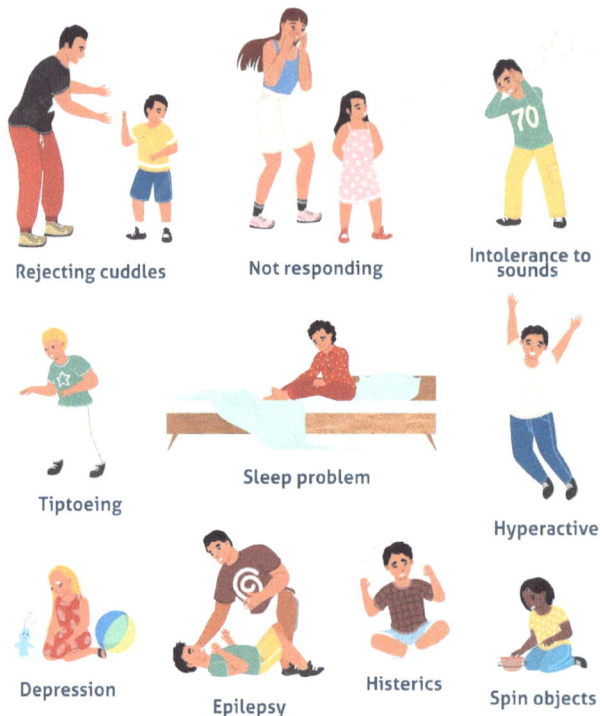

Autism has many problems not answering, not paying attention, not like loud sound, sleep disorder, hyperactive, repetitive, spin or throw objects, many sensitives by brain, head banging, and depression.

https://effectivehealthcare.ahrq.gov/products/autism-update/consumer

All ADHD, Autism, and depression are treatable through better living, improving behaviors, education, therapies, and the most important is medicine.

- Behavioral management therapy
- Cognitive behavior therapy
- Early intervention
- Educational and school-based therapies
- Joint attention therapy
- Medication treatment
- Nutritional therapy
- Occupational therapy
- Parent-mediated therapy
- Physical therapy
- Social skills training
- Speech-language therapy

https://www.nichd.nih.gov/health/topics/autism/conditioninfo/treatments

Parents should consult and request the doctor for the kid to attend the therapies. Each kid may need one or more therapies. Therapies may help, but may not work without the medicine because ADHD, autism, depression are caused by brain disorders.

ADHD Medications

	Brand Name	FDA Approved
Stimulants		
Short-acting amphetamine	Adderall, Dexedrine, Detrostat	Yes
Short-acting methylphenidate	Focalin, Methylin, Ritalin	Yes
Intermediate-acting methylphenidate	Metadate CD, Ritalin LA	Yes
Long-acting amphetamine	Adderall-XR, Dexedrine Spansule, Vyvanse	Yes
Long-acting methylphenidate	Concerta, Daytrana, Focalin XR, Quillivant XR	Yes
Non-Stimulants		
Atomoxetine	Strattera	Yes
Guanfacine	Intuniv (long-acting); Tenex (short-acting)	Yes
Clonidine	Kapvay	Yes
Bupropion	Wellbutrin	No

https://www.madinamerica.com/adhd-info/

By the age of six, my son started taking guanfacine and then methylphenidate. It may not work for everyone or long. It was working for my kid for about 2 months, then it stopped working. I created a model as the cover page showing him having depression.

ADHD Medication: Non-stimulants

Class	Generic Name	Brand Name	Duration
SELECTIVE NOREPINEPHRINE REUPTAKE INHIBITOR	atomoxetine hydrochloride	Strattera®	24 hours
	viloxazine	Qelbree™	24 hours
ALPHA-2 ADRENERGIC AGONIST	clonidine hydrochloride	Kapvay®	12 to 24 hours
	guanfacine hydrochloride	Intuniv®	12 to 24 hours

Cleveland Clinic

https://my.clevelandclinic.org/health/treatments/11766-adhd-medication

It is important to know the medicines. It may take some time to weeks for the medicine to work. Suddenly stopping taking the medicines may be worse. Ask the doctor.

FDA-approved antidepressants for children and teenagers

Medication*	Age (in years)	Diagnosis
Clomipramine (Anafranil)	10 and older	Obsessive-compulsive disorder (OCD)
Duloxetine (Cymbalta, Drizalma Sprinkle)	7 and older	Generalized anxiety disorder
Escitalopram (Lexapro)	12 and older	Major depressive disorder
Fluoxetine (Prozac)	8 and older	Major depressive disorder
	7 and older	OCD
Fluvoxamine	8 and older	OCD
Lurasidone (Latuda)	10 and older	Bipolar depression
Olanzapine and fluoxetine, combination drug (Symbyax)	10 and older	Bipolar depression
Sertraline (Zoloft)	6 and older	OCD

*Many of these drugs are also available in generic form. Recommended initial dose and maximum dose vary by age.

https://www.mayoclinic.org/diseases-conditions/teen-depression/in-depth/antidepressants/art-20047502

Depression may be caused by chemical imbalance. Serotonin is the main chemical to regulate the brain. The two popular drugs are Escitalopram (Lexapro) and Zoloft are belong to the group called selective serotonin reuptake inhibitors (SSRI)

The serotonin

The serotonin chemical controls the brain's functions and behaviors. Low serotonin causes many brain problems. The study shows that supplementation with omega-3 fatty acids and vitamin D increase serotonin.

https://pubmed.ncbi.nlm.nih.gov/25713056/

https://www.verywellmind.com/what-is-serotonin-425327

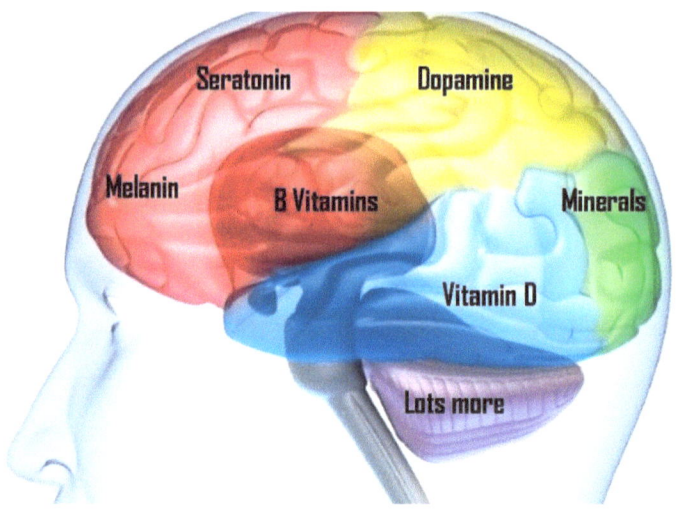

https://www.cmbhealthspecialties.com/brain-health

the three Brains chemicals associate with ADHD, Autism, and depression are serotonin, dopamine, and

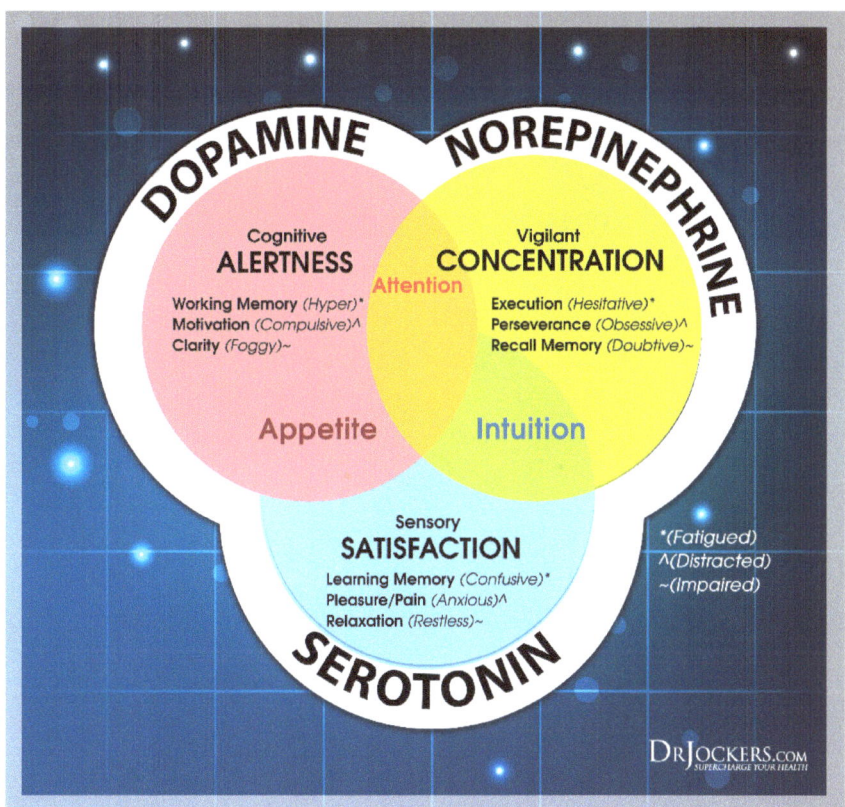

Dopamine and Norepinephrine are associated with ADHD, and Serotonin associated with anxieties and depression.

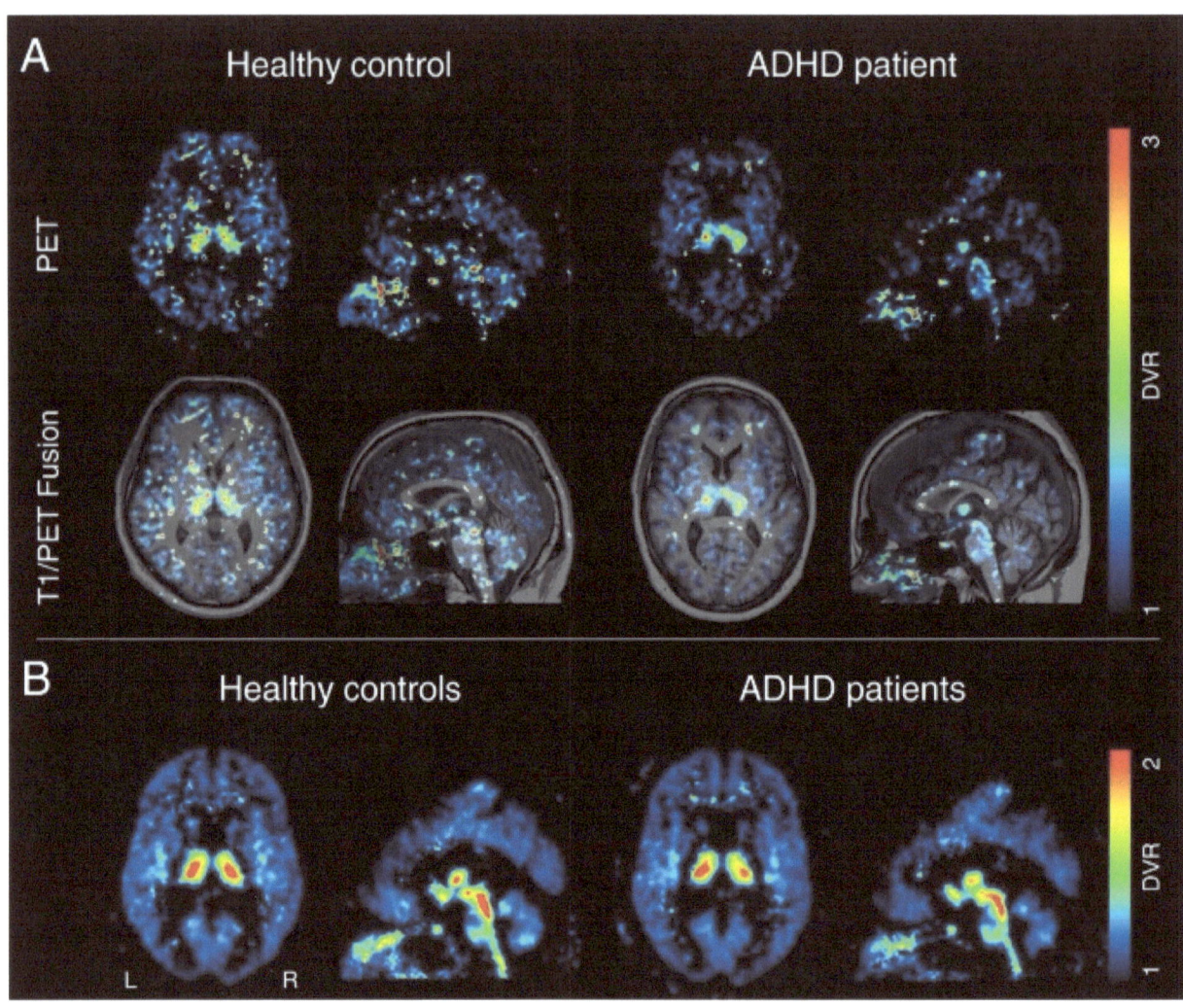

https://www.nature.com/articles/s41398-019-0619-y#Fig1

The images show the brain's activities. The brain controls the behaviors. Thus, the brain needs medical treatment for all ADHD, autism, and depression.

In my theory and experience, depression needs to be cured first, then ADHD. If the person takes both medicines to treat ADHD and depression, it may cause an overdose of serotonin or other chemicals in the brain even if it is rarely to happen but may be very dangerous.

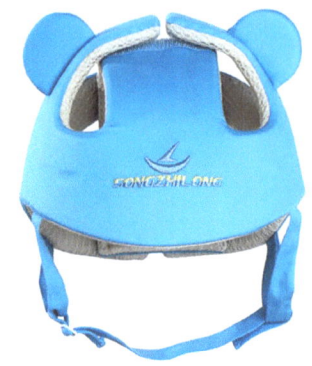

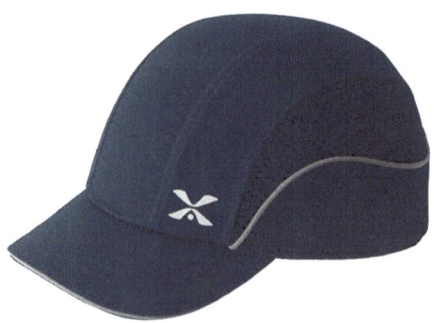

Helmets are used to help kids from head injuries in school and at home. I had tried many on Amazon.

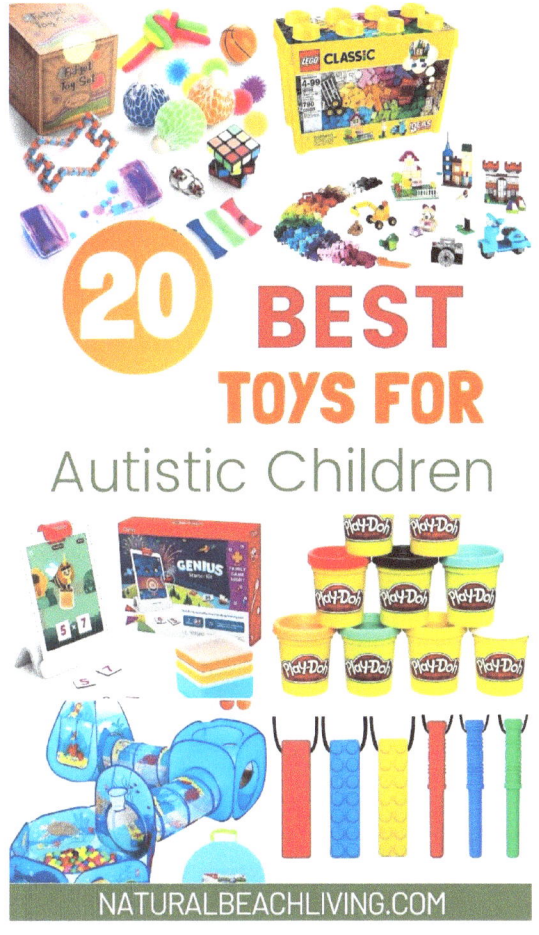

Stem toys are used in therapies to teach autism. There are tons of toys on Amazon. I spent over one thousand dollars.

Things to do for Autism.

Take medicine.

Playing Legos
Basic video games
Swimming
Puzzle Solving
Riding Bikes
Visiting Places
Outdoor Activities
Game Centers
Exercises
Music

Things NOT to do with Autism.

Do not use drugs on the counter.
NOT too much time on screen
Do not eat salty food.
Do not eat sweat food.
NO Jumping
NO Running

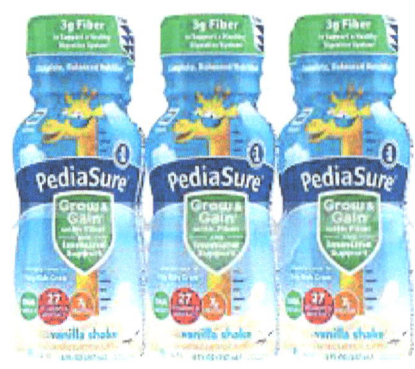

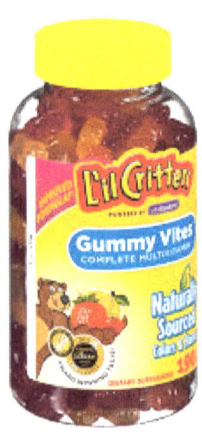

Nutrition

Autism children are sensitive to food even with multivitamins and other supplement milks. It takes many tries for them to like it. So, keep trying…They may not like the sugar coat and skin rash with vanilla.

I have been researching ADHD, autism, and depression for two years since these disorders are complex. I started learning my son's behaviors, visualizing his brain, creating the cycle of the three disorders, and learning the medicines for treatments.

In conclusion with one line writing, the combination of therapies and medicines are the best treatments.

Other References

https://www.cdc.gov/ncbddd/autism/signs.html

https://www.autismspeaks.org/what-autism

https://childmind.org/guide/autism-spectrum-disorder-quick-guide/

https://www.nichd.nih.gov/health/topics/autism/conditioninfo/treatments/medication-treatment

https://www.mayoclinic.org/diseases-conditions/teen-depression/in-depth/antidepressants/art-20047502

https://www.cdc.gov/ncbddd/adhd/conditions.html

https://www.webmd.com/add-adhd/childhood-adhd/adhd-treatment-overview